THIS BOOK BELONGS TO :

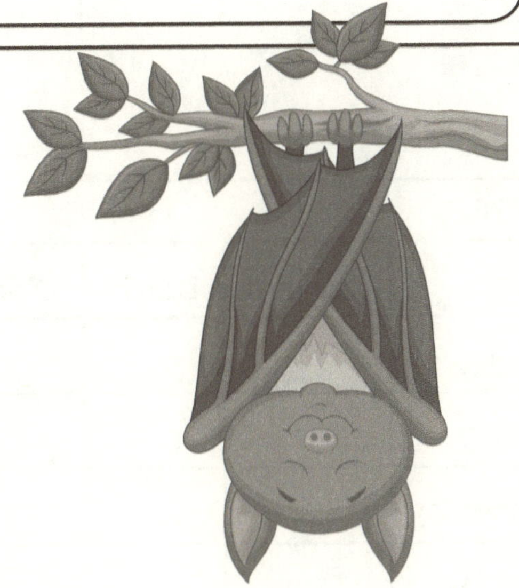

SUGAR MONITOR

DATE						
DAY	Breakfast	Lunch	Dinner	Snack	Bedtime	Other
Monday						
Tuesday						
Wednesday						
Thursday						
Friday						
Saturday						
Sunday						

DATE						
DAY	Breakfast	Lunch	Dinner	Snack	Bedtime	Other
Monday						
Tuesday						
Wednesday						
Thursday						
Friday						
Saturday						
Sunday						

SUGAR MONITOR

DATE						
DAY	Breakfast	Lunch	Dinner	Snack	Bedtime	Other
Monday						
Tuesday						
Wednesday						
Thursday						
Friday						
Saturday						
Sunday						

DATE						
DAY	Breakfast	Lunch	Dinner	Snack	Bedtime	Other
Monday						
Tuesday						
Wednesday						
Thursday						
Friday						
Saturday						
Sunday						

SUGAR MONITOR

DATE						
DAY	Breakfast	Lunch	Dinner	Snack	Bedtime	Other
Monday						
Tuesday						
Wednesday						
Thursday						
Friday						
Saturday						
Sunday						

DATE						
DAY	Breakfast	Lunch	Dinner	Snack	Bedtime	Other
Monday						
Tuesday						
Wednesday						
Thursday						
Friday						
Saturday						
Sunday						

SUGAR MONITOR

DATE						
DAY	Breakfast	Lunch	Dinner	Snack	Bedtime	Other
Monday						
Tuesday						
Wednesday						
Thursday						
Friday						
Saturday						
Sunday						

DATE						
DAY	Breakfast	Lunch	Dinner	Snack	Bedtime	Other
Monday						
Tuesday						
Wednesday						
Thursday						
Friday						
Saturday						
Sunday						

SUGAR MONITOR

DATE						
DAY	Breakfast	Lunch	Dinner	Snack	Bedtime	Other
Monday						
Tuesday						
Wednesday						
Thursday						
Friday						
Saturday						
Sunday						

DATE						
DAY	Breakfast	Lunch	Dinner	Snack	Bedtime	Other
Monday						
Tuesday						
Wednesday						
Thursday						
Friday						
Saturday						
Sunday						

SUGAR MONITOR

DATE						
DAY	Breakfast	Lunch	Dinner	Snack	Bedtime	Other
Monday						
Tuesday						
Wednesday						
Thursday						
Friday						
Saturday						
Sunday						

DATE						
DAY	Breakfast	Lunch	Dinner	Snack	Bedtime	Other
Monday						
Tuesday						
Wednesday						
Thursday						
Friday						
Saturday						
Sunday						

SUGAR MONITOR

DATE						
DAY	Breakfast	Lunch	Dinner	Snack	Bedtime	Other
Monday						
Tuesday						
Wednesday						
Thursday						
Friday						
Saturday						
Sunday						

DATE						
DAY	Breakfast	Lunch	Dinner	Snack	Bedtime	Other
Monday						
Tuesday						
Wednesday						
Thursday						
Friday						
Saturday						
Sunday						

SUGAR MONITOR

DATE						
DAY	Breakfast	Lunch	Dinner	Snack	Bedtime	Other
Monday						
Tuesday						
Wednesday						
Thursday						
Friday						
Saturday						
Sunday						

DATE						
DAY	Breakfast	Lunch	Dinner	Snack	Bedtime	Other
Monday						
Tuesday						
Wednesday						
Thursday						
Friday						
Saturday						
Sunday						

SUGAR MONITOR

DATE						
DAY	Breakfast	Lunch	Dinner	Snack	Bedtime	Other
Monday						
Tuesday						
Wednesday						
Thursday						
Friday						
Saturday						
Sunday						

DATE						
DAY	Breakfast	Lunch	Dinner	Snack	Bedtime	Other
Monday						
Tuesday						
Wednesday						
Thursday						
Friday						
Saturday						
Sunday						

SUGAR MONITOR

DATE						
DAY	Breakfast	Lunch	Dinner	Snack	Bedtime	Other
Monday						
Tuesday						
Wednesday						
Thursday						
Friday						
Saturday						
Sunday						

DATE						
DAY	Breakfast	Lunch	Dinner	Snack	Bedtime	Other
Monday						
Tuesday						
Wednesday						
Thursday						
Friday						
Saturday						
Sunday						

SUGAR MONITOR

DATE						
DAY	Breakfast	Lunch	Dinner	Snack	Bedtime	Other
Monday						
Tuesday						
Wednesday						
Thursday						
Friday						
Saturday						
Sunday						

DATE						
DAY	Breakfast	Lunch	Dinner	Snack	Bedtime	Other
Monday						
Tuesday						
Wednesday						
Thursday						
Friday						
Saturday						
Sunday						

SUGAR MONITOR

DATE						
DAY	Breakfast	Lunch	Dinner	Snack	Bedtime	Other
Monday						
Tuesday						
Wednesday						
Thursday						
Friday						
Saturday						
Sunday						

DATE						
DAY	Breakfast	Lunch	Dinner	Snack	Bedtime	Other
Monday						
Tuesday						
Wednesday						
Thursday						
Friday						
Saturday						
Sunday						

SUGAR MONITOR

DATE						
DAY	Breakfast	Lunch	Dinner	Snack	Bedtime	Other
Monday						
Tuesday						
Wednesday						
Thursday						
Friday						
Saturday						
Sunday						

DATE						
DAY	Breakfast	Lunch	Dinner	Snack	Bedtime	Other
Monday						
Tuesday						
Wednesday						
Thursday						
Friday						
Saturday						
Sunday						

SUGAR MONITOR

DATE						
DAY	Breakfast	Lunch	Dinner	Snack	Bedtime	Other
Monday						
Tuesday						
Wednesday						
Thursday						
Friday						
Saturday						
Sunday						

DATE						
DAY	Breakfast	Lunch	Dinner	Snack	Bedtime	Other
Monday						
Tuesday						
Wednesday						
Thursday						
Friday						
Saturday						
Sunday						

SUGAR MONITOR

DATE						
DAY	Breakfast	Lunch	Dinner	Snack	Bedtime	Other
Monday						
Tuesday						
Wednesday						
Thursday						
Friday						
Saturday						
Sunday						

DATE						
DAY	Breakfast	Lunch	Dinner	Snack	Bedtime	Other
Monday						
Tuesday						
Wednesday						
Thursday						
Friday						
Saturday						
Sunday						

SUGAR MONITOR

DATE						
DAY	Breakfast	Lunch	Dinner	Snack	Bedtime	Other
Monday						
Tuesday						
Wednesday						
Thursday						
Friday						
Saturday						
Sunday						

DATE						
DAY	Breakfast	Lunch	Dinner	Snack	Bedtime	Other
Monday						
Tuesday						
Wednesday						
Thursday						
Friday						
Saturday						
Sunday						

SUGAR MONITOR

DATE						
DAY	Breakfast	Lunch	Dinner	Snack	Bedtime	Other
Monday						
Tuesday						
Wednesday						
Thursday						
Friday						
Saturday						
Sunday						

DATE						
DAY	Breakfast	Lunch	Dinner	Snack	Bedtime	Other
Monday						
Tuesday						
Wednesday						
Thursday						
Friday						
Saturday						
Sunday						

SUGAR MONITOR

DATE						
DAY	Breakfast	Lunch	Dinner	Snack	Bedtime	Other
Monday						
Tuesday						
Wednesday						
Thursday						
Friday						
Saturday						
Sunday						

DATE						
DAY	Breakfast	Lunch	Dinner	Snack	Bedtime	Other
Monday						
Tuesday						
Wednesday						
Thursday						
Friday						
Saturday						
Sunday						

SUGAR MONITOR

DATE						
DAY	Breakfast	Lunch	Dinner	Snack	Bedtime	Other
Monday						
Tuesday						
Wednesday						
Thursday						
Friday						
Saturday						
Sunday						

DATE						
DAY	Breakfast	Lunch	Dinner	Snack	Bedtime	Other
Monday						
Tuesday						
Wednesday						
Thursday						
Friday						
Saturday						
Sunday						

SUGAR MONITOR

DATE						
DAY	Breakfast	Lunch	Dinner	Snack	Bedtime	Other
Monday						
Tuesday						
Wednesday						
Thursday						
Friday						
Saturday						
Sunday						

DATE						
DAY	Breakfast	Lunch	Dinner	Snack	Bedtime	Other
Monday						
Tuesday						
Wednesday						
Thursday						
Friday						
Saturday						
Sunday						

SUGAR MONITOR

DATE						
DAY	Breakfast	Lunch	Dinner	Snack	Bedtime	Other
Monday						
Tuesday						
Wednesday						
Thursday						
Friday						
Saturday						
Sunday						

DATE						
DAY	Breakfast	Lunch	Dinner	Snack	Bedtime	Other
Monday						
Tuesday						
Wednesday						
Thursday						
Friday						
Saturday						
Sunday						

SUGAR MONITOR

DATE						
DAY	Breakfast	Lunch	Dinner	Snack	Bedtime	Other
Monday						
Tuesday						
Wednesday						
Thursday						
Friday						
Saturday						
Sunday						

DATE						
DAY	Breakfast	Lunch	Dinner	Snack	Bedtime	Other
Monday						
Tuesday						
Wednesday						
Thursday						
Friday						
Saturday						
Sunday						

SUGAR MONITOR

DATE						
DAY	Breakfast	Lunch	Dinner	Snack	Bedtime	Other
Monday						
Tuesday						
Wednesday						
Thursday						
Friday						
Saturday						
Sunday						

DATE						
DAY	Breakfast	Lunch	Dinner	Snack	Bedtime	Other
Monday						
Tuesday						
Wednesday						
Thursday						
Friday						
Saturday						
Sunday						

SUGAR MONITOR

DATE						
DAY	Breakfast	Lunch	Dinner	Snack	Bedtime	Other
Monday						
Tuesday						
Wednesday						
Thursday						
Friday						
Saturday						
Sunday						

DATE						
DAY	Breakfast	Lunch	Dinner	Snack	Bedtime	Other
Monday						
Tuesday						
Wednesday						
Thursday						
Friday						
Saturday						
Sunday						

SUGAR MONITOR

DATE						
DAY	Breakfast	Lunch	Dinner	Snack	Bedtime	Other
Monday						
Tuesday						
Wednesday						
Thursday						
Friday						
Saturday						
Sunday						

DATE						
DAY	Breakfast	Lunch	Dinner	Snack	Bedtime	Other
Monday						
Tuesday						
Wednesday						
Thursday						
Friday						
Saturday						
Sunday						

SUGAR MONITOR

DATE						
DAY	Breakfast	Lunch	Dinner	Snack	Bedtime	Other
Monday						
Tuesday						
Wednesday						
Thursday						
Friday						
Saturday						
Sunday						

DATE						
DAY	Breakfast	Lunch	Dinner	Snack	Bedtime	Other
Monday						
Tuesday						
Wednesday						
Thursday						
Friday						
Saturday						
Sunday						

SUGAR MONITOR

DATE						
DAY	Breakfast	Lunch	Dinner	Snack	Bedtime	Other
Monday						
Tuesday						
Wednesday						
Thursday						
Friday						
Saturday						
Sunday						

DATE						
DAY	Breakfast	Lunch	Dinner	Snack	Bedtime	Other
Monday						
Tuesday						
Wednesday						
Thursday						
Friday						
Saturday						
Sunday						

SUGAR MONITOR

DATE						
DAY	Breakfast	Lunch	Dinner	Snack	Bedtime	Other
Monday						
Tuesday						
Wednesday						
Thursday						
Friday						
Saturday						
Sunday						

DATE						
DAY	Breakfast	Lunch	Dinner	Snack	Bedtime	Other
Monday						
Tuesday						
Wednesday						
Thursday						
Friday						
Saturday						
Sunday						

SUGAR MONITOR

DATE						
DAY	Breakfast	Lunch	Dinner	Snack	Bedtime	Other
Monday						
Tuesday						
Wednesday						
Thursday						
Friday						
Saturday						
Sunday						

DATE						
DAY	Breakfast	Lunch	Dinner	Snack	Bedtime	Other
Monday						
Tuesday						
Wednesday						
Thursday						
Friday						
Saturday						
Sunday						

SUGAR MONITOR

DATE						
DAY	Breakfast	Lunch	Dinner	Snack	Bedtime	Other
Monday						
Tuesday						
Wednesday						
Thursday						
Friday						
Saturday						
Sunday						

DATE						
DAY	Breakfast	Lunch	Dinner	Snack	Bedtime	Other
Monday						
Tuesday						
Wednesday						
Thursday						
Friday						
Saturday						
Sunday						

SUGAR MONITOR

DATE						
DAY	Breakfast	Lunch	Dinner	Snack	Bedtime	Other
Monday						
Tuesday						
Wednesday						
Thursday						
Friday						
Saturday						
Sunday						

DATE						
DAY	Breakfast	Lunch	Dinner	Snack	Bedtime	Other
Monday						
Tuesday						
Wednesday						
Thursday						
Friday						
Saturday						
Sunday						

SUGAR MONITOR

DATE						
DAY	Breakfast	Lunch	Dinner	Snack	Bedtime	Other
Monday						
Tuesday						
Wednesday						
Thursday						
Friday						
Saturday						
Sunday						

DATE						
DAY	Breakfast	Lunch	Dinner	Snack	Bedtime	Other
Monday						
Tuesday						
Wednesday						
Thursday						
Friday						
Saturday						
Sunday						

SUGAR MONITOR

DATE						
DAY	Breakfast	Lunch	Dinner	Snack	Bedtime	Other
Monday						
Tuesday						
Wednesday						
Thursday						
Friday						
Saturday						
Sunday						

DATE						
DAY	Breakfast	Lunch	Dinner	Snack	Bedtime	Other
Monday						
Tuesday						
Wednesday						
Thursday						
Friday						
Saturday						
Sunday						

SUGAR MONITOR

DATE						
DAY	Breakfast	Lunch	Dinner	Snack	Bedtime	Other
Monday						
Tuesday						
Wednesday						
Thursday						
Friday						
Saturday						
Sunday						

DATE						
DAY	Breakfast	Lunch	Dinner	Snack	Bedtime	Other
Monday						
Tuesday						
Wednesday						
Thursday						
Friday						
Saturday						
Sunday						

SUGAR MONITOR

DATE						
DAY	Breakfast	Lunch	Dinner	Snack	Bedtime	Other
Monday						
Tuesday						
Wednesday						
Thursday						
Friday						
Saturday						
Sunday						

DATE						
DAY	Breakfast	Lunch	Dinner	Snack	Bedtime	Other
Monday						
Tuesday						
Wednesday						
Thursday						
Friday						
Saturday						
Sunday						

SUGAR MONITOR

DATE						
DAY	Breakfast	Lunch	Dinner	Snack	Bedtime	Other
Monday						
Tuesday						
Wednesday						
Thursday						
Friday						
Saturday						
Sunday						

DATE						
DAY	Breakfast	Lunch	Dinner	Snack	Bedtime	Other
Monday						
Tuesday						
Wednesday						
Thursday						
Friday						
Saturday						
Sunday						

SUGAR MONITOR

DATE						
DAY	Breakfast	Lunch	Dinner	Snack	Bedtime	Other
Monday						
Tuesday						
Wednesday						
Thursday						
Friday						
Saturday						
Sunday						

DATE						
DAY	Breakfast	Lunch	Dinner	Snack	Bedtime	Other
Monday						
Tuesday						
Wednesday						
Thursday						
Friday						
Saturday						
Sunday						

SUGAR MONITOR

DATE						
DAY	Breakfast	Lunch	Dinner	Snack	Bedtime	Other
Monday						
Tuesday						
Wednesday						
Thursday						
Friday						
Saturday						
Sunday						

DATE						
DAY	Breakfast	Lunch	Dinner	Snack	Bedtime	Other
Monday						
Tuesday						
Wednesday						
Thursday						
Friday						
Saturday						
Sunday						

SUGAR MONITOR

DATE						
DAY	Breakfast	Lunch	Dinner	Snack	Bedtime	Other
Monday						
Tuesday						
Wednesday						
Thursday						
Friday						
Saturday						
Sunday						

DATE						
DAY	Breakfast	Lunch	Dinner	Snack	Bedtime	Other
Monday						
Tuesday						
Wednesday						
Thursday						
Friday						
Saturday						
Sunday						

SUGAR MONITOR

DATE						
DAY	Breakfast	Lunch	Dinner	Snack	Bedtime	Other
Monday						
Tuesday						
Wednesday						
Thursday						
Friday						
Saturday						
Sunday						

DATE						
DAY	Breakfast	Lunch	Dinner	Snack	Bedtime	Other
Monday						
Tuesday						
Wednesday						
Thursday						
Friday						
Saturday						
Sunday						

SUGAR MONITOR

DATE						
DAY	Breakfast	Lunch	Dinner	Snack	Bedtime	Other
Monday						
Tuesday						
Wednesday						
Thursday						
Friday						
Saturday						
Sunday						

DATE						
DAY	Breakfast	Lunch	Dinner	Snack	Bedtime	Other
Monday						
Tuesday						
Wednesday						
Thursday						
Friday						
Saturday						
Sunday						

SUGAR MONITOR

DATE						
DAY	Breakfast	Lunch	Dinner	Snack	Bedtime	Other
Monday						
Tuesday						
Wednesday						
Thursday						
Friday						
Saturday						
Sunday						

DATE						
DAY	Breakfast	Lunch	Dinner	Snack	Bedtime	Other
Monday						
Tuesday						
Wednesday						
Thursday						
Friday						
Saturday						
Sunday						

SUGAR MONITOR

DATE						
DAY	Breakfast	Lunch	Dinner	Snack	Bedtime	Other
Monday						
Tuesday						
Wednesday						
Thursday						
Friday						
Saturday						
Sunday						

DATE						
DAY	Breakfast	Lunch	Dinner	Snack	Bedtime	Other
Monday						
Tuesday						
Wednesday						
Thursday						
Friday						
Saturday						
Sunday						

SUGAR MONITOR

DATE						
DAY	Breakfast	Lunch	Dinner	Snack	Bedtime	Other
Monday						
Tuesday						
Wednesday						
Thursday						
Friday						
Saturday						
Sunday						

DATE						
DAY	Breakfast	Lunch	Dinner	Snack	Bedtime	Other
Monday						
Tuesday						
Wednesday						
Thursday						
Friday						
Saturday						
Sunday						

SUGAR MONITOR

DATE						
DAY	Breakfast	Lunch	Dinner	Snack	Bedtime	Other
Monday						
Tuesday						
Wednesday						
Thursday						
Friday						
Saturday						
Sunday						

DATE						
DAY	Breakfast	Lunch	Dinner	Snack	Bedtime	Other
Monday						
Tuesday						
Wednesday						
Thursday						
Friday						
Saturday						
Sunday						

SUGAR MONITOR

DATE						
DAY	Breakfast	Lunch	Dinner	Snack	Bedtime	Other
Monday						
Tuesday						
Wednesday						
Thursday						
Friday						
Saturday						
Sunday						

DATE						
DAY	Breakfast	Lunch	Dinner	Snack	Bedtime	Other
Monday						
Tuesday						
Wednesday						
Thursday						
Friday						
Saturday						
Sunday						

SUGAR MONITOR

DATE						
DAY	Breakfast	Lunch	Dinner	Snack	Bedtime	Other
Monday						
Tuesday						
Wednesday						
Thursday						
Friday						
Saturday						
Sunday						

DATE						
DAY	Breakfast	Lunch	Dinner	Snack	Bedtime	Other
Monday						
Tuesday						
Wednesday						
Thursday						
Friday						
Saturday						
Sunday						

SUGAR MONITOR

DATE						
DAY	Breakfast	Lunch	Dinner	Snack	Bedtime	Other
Monday						
Tuesday						
Wednesday						
Thursday						
Friday						
Saturday						
Sunday						

DATE						
DAY	Breakfast	Lunch	Dinner	Snack	Bedtime	Other
Monday						
Tuesday						
Wednesday						
Thursday						
Friday						
Saturday						
Sunday						

SUGAR MONITOR

DATE						
DAY	Breakfast	Lunch	Dinner	Snack	Bedtime	Other
Monday						
Tuesday						
Wednesday						
Thursday						
Friday						
Saturday						
Sunday						

DATE						
DAY	Breakfast	Lunch	Dinner	Snack	Bedtime	Other
Monday						
Tuesday						
Wednesday						
Thursday						
Friday						
Saturday						
Sunday						

SUGAR MONITOR

DATE						
DAY	Breakfast	Lunch	Dinner	Snack	Bedtime	Other
Monday						
Tuesday						
Wednesday						
Thursday						
Friday						
Saturday						
Sunday						

DATE						
DAY	Breakfast	Lunch	Dinner	Snack	Bedtime	Other
Monday						
Tuesday						
Wednesday						
Thursday						
Friday						
Saturday						
Sunday						

SUGAR MONITOR

DATE						
DAY	Breakfast	Lunch	Dinner	Snack	Bedtime	Other
Monday						
Tuesday						
Wednesday						
Thursday						
Friday						
Saturday						
Sunday						

DATE						
DAY	Breakfast	Lunch	Dinner	Snack	Bedtime	Other
Monday						
Tuesday						
Wednesday						
Thursday						
Friday						
Saturday						
Sunday						

SUGAR MONITOR

DATE						
DAY	Breakfast	Lunch	Dinner	Snack	Bedtime	Other
Monday						
Tuesday						
Wednesday						
Thursday						
Friday						
Saturday						
Sunday						

DATE						
DAY	Breakfast	Lunch	Dinner	Snack	Bedtime	Other
Monday						
Tuesday						
Wednesday						
Thursday						
Friday						
Saturday						
Sunday						

SUGAR MONITOR

DATE						
DAY	Breakfast	Lunch	Dinner	Snack	Bedtime	Other
Monday						
Tuesday						
Wednesday						
Thursday						
Friday						
Saturday						
Sunday						

DATE						
DAY	Breakfast	Lunch	Dinner	Snack	Bedtime	Other
Monday						
Tuesday						
Wednesday						
Thursday						
Friday						
Saturday						
Sunday						

SUGAR MONITOR

DATE						
DAY	Breakfast	Lunch	Dinner	Snack	Bedtime	Other
Monday						
Tuesday						
Wednesday						
Thursday						
Friday						
Saturday						
Sunday						

DATE						
DAY	Breakfast	Lunch	Dinner	Snack	Bedtime	Other
Monday						
Tuesday						
Wednesday						
Thursday						
Friday						
Saturday						
Sunday						

SUGAR MONITOR

DATE						
DAY	Breakfast	Lunch	Dinner	Snack	Bedtime	Other
Monday						
Tuesday						
Wednesday						
Thursday						
Friday						
Saturday						
Sunday						

DATE						
DAY	Breakfast	Lunch	Dinner	Snack	Bedtime	Other
Monday						
Tuesday						
Wednesday						
Thursday						
Friday						
Saturday						
Sunday						

SUGAR MONITOR

DATE						
DAY	Breakfast	Lunch	Dinner	Snack	Bedtime	Other
Monday						
Tuesday						
Wednesday						
Thursday						
Friday						
Saturday						
Sunday						

DATE						
DAY	Breakfast	Lunch	Dinner	Snack	Bedtime	Other
Monday						
Tuesday						
Wednesday						
Thursday						
Friday						
Saturday						
Sunday						

SUGAR MONITOR

DATE						
DAY	Breakfast	Lunch	Dinner	Snack	Bedtime	Other
Monday						
Tuesday						
Wednesday						
Thursday						
Friday						
Saturday						
Sunday						

DATE						
DAY	Breakfast	Lunch	Dinner	Snack	Bedtime	Other
Monday						
Tuesday						
Wednesday						
Thursday						
Friday						
Saturday						
Sunday						

SUGAR MONITOR

DATE						
DAY	Breakfast	Lunch	Dinner	Snack	Bedtime	Other
Monday						
Tuesday						
Wednesday						
Thursday						
Friday						
Saturday						
Sunday						

DATE						
DAY	Breakfast	Lunch	Dinner	Snack	Bedtime	Other
Monday						
Tuesday						
Wednesday						
Thursday						
Friday						
Saturday						
Sunday						

SUGAR MONITOR

DATE						
DAY	Breakfast	Lunch	Dinner	Snack	Bedtime	Other
Monday						
Tuesday						
Wednesday						
Thursday						
Friday						
Saturday						
Sunday						

DATE						
DAY	Breakfast	Lunch	Dinner	Snack	Bedtime	Other
Monday						
Tuesday						
Wednesday						
Thursday						
Friday						
Saturday						
Sunday						

SUGAR MONITOR

DATE						
DAY	Breakfast	Lunch	Dinner	Snack	Bedtime	Other
Monday						
Tuesday						
Wednesday						
Thursday						
Friday						
Saturday						
Sunday						

DATE						
DAY	Breakfast	Lunch	Dinner	Snack	Bedtime	Other
Monday						
Tuesday						
Wednesday						
Thursday						
Friday						
Saturday						
Sunday						

SUGAR MONITOR

DATE						
DAY	Breakfast	Lunch	Dinner	Snack	Bedtime	Other
Monday						
Tuesday						
Wednesday						
Thursday						
Friday						
Saturday						
Sunday						

DATE						
DAY	Breakfast	Lunch	Dinner	Snack	Bedtime	Other
Monday						
Tuesday						
Wednesday						
Thursday						
Friday						
Saturday						
Sunday						

SUGAR MONITOR

DATE						
DAY	Breakfast	Lunch	Dinner	Snack	Bedtime	Other
Monday						
Tuesday						
Wednesday						
Thursday						
Friday						
Saturday						
Sunday						

DATE						
DAY	Breakfast	Lunch	Dinner	Snack	Bedtime	Other
Monday						
Tuesday						
Wednesday						
Thursday						
Friday						
Saturday						
Sunday						

SUGAR MONITOR

DATE						
DAY	Breakfast	Lunch	Dinner	Snack	Bedtime	Other
Monday						
Tuesday						
Wednesday						
Thursday						
Friday						
Saturday						
Sunday						

DATE						
DAY	Breakfast	Lunch	Dinner	Snack	Bedtime	Other
Monday						
Tuesday						
Wednesday						
Thursday						
Friday						
Saturday						
Sunday						

SUGAR MONITOR

DATE						
DAY	Breakfast	Lunch	Dinner	Snack	Bedtime	Other
Monday						
Tuesday						
Wednesday						
Thursday						
Friday						
Saturday						
Sunday						

DATE						
DAY	Breakfast	Lunch	Dinner	Snack	Bedtime	Other
Monday						
Tuesday						
Wednesday						
Thursday						
Friday						
Saturday						
Sunday						

SUGAR MONITOR

DATE						
DAY	Breakfast	Lunch	Dinner	Snack	Bedtime	Other
Monday						
Tuesday						
Wednesday						
Thursday						
Friday						
Saturday						
Sunday						

DATE						
DAY	Breakfast	Lunch	Dinner	Snack	Bedtime	Other
Monday						
Tuesday						
Wednesday						
Thursday						
Friday						
Saturday						
Sunday						

SUGAR MONITOR

DATE						
DAY	Breakfast	Lunch	Dinner	Snack	Bedtime	Other
Monday						
Tuesday						
Wednesday						
Thursday						
Friday						
Saturday						
Sunday						

DATE						
DAY	Breakfast	Lunch	Dinner	Snack	Bedtime	Other
Monday						
Tuesday						
Wednesday						
Thursday						
Friday						
Saturday						
Sunday						

SUGAR MONITOR

DATE						
DAY	Breakfast	Lunch	Dinner	Snack	Bedtime	Other
Monday						
Tuesday						
Wednesday						
Thursday						
Friday						
Saturday						
Sunday						

DATE						
DAY	Breakfast	Lunch	Dinner	Snack	Bedtime	Other
Monday						
Tuesday						
Wednesday						
Thursday						
Friday						
Saturday						
Sunday						

SUGAR MONITOR

DATE						
DAY	Breakfast	Lunch	Dinner	Snack	Bedtime	Other
Monday						
Tuesday						
Wednesday						
Thursday						
Friday						
Saturday						
Sunday						

DATE						
DAY	Breakfast	Lunch	Dinner	Snack	Bedtime	Other
Monday						
Tuesday						
Wednesday						
Thursday						
Friday						
Saturday						
Sunday						

SUGAR MONITOR

DATE						
DAY	Breakfast	Lunch	Dinner	Snack	Bedtime	Other
Monday						
Tuesday						
Wednesday						
Thursday						
Friday						
Saturday						
Sunday						

DATE						
DAY	Breakfast	Lunch	Dinner	Snack	Bedtime	Other
Monday						
Tuesday						
Wednesday						
Thursday						
Friday						
Saturday						
Sunday						

SUGAR MONITOR

DATE						
DAY	Breakfast	Lunch	Dinner	Snack	Bedtime	Other
Monday						
Tuesday						
Wednesday						
Thursday						
Friday						
Saturday						
Sunday						

DATE						
DAY	Breakfast	Lunch	Dinner	Snack	Bedtime	Other
Monday						
Tuesday						
Wednesday						
Thursday						
Friday						
Saturday						
Sunday						

SUGAR MONITOR

DATE						
DAY	Breakfast	Lunch	Dinner	Snack	Bedtime	Other
Monday						
Tuesday						
Wednesday						
Thursday						
Friday						
Saturday						
Sunday						

DATE						
DAY	Breakfast	Lunch	Dinner	Snack	Bedtime	Other
Monday						
Tuesday						
Wednesday						
Thursday						
Friday						
Saturday						
Sunday						

SUGAR MONITOR

DATE						
DAY	Breakfast	Lunch	Dinner	Snack	Bedtime	Other
Monday						
Tuesday						
Wednesday						
Thursday						
Friday						
Saturday						
Sunday						

DATE						
DAY	Breakfast	Lunch	Dinner	Snack	Bedtime	Other
Monday						
Tuesday						
Wednesday						
Thursday						
Friday						
Saturday						
Sunday						

SUGAR MONITOR

DATE						
DAY	Breakfast	Lunch	Dinner	Snack	Bedtime	Other
Monday						
Tuesday						
Wednesday						
Thursday						
Friday						
Saturday						
Sunday						

DATE						
DAY	Breakfast	Lunch	Dinner	Snack	Bedtime	Other
Monday						
Tuesday						
Wednesday						
Thursday						
Friday						
Saturday						
Sunday						

SUGAR MONITOR

DATE						
DAY	Breakfast	Lunch	Dinner	Snack	Bedtime	Other
Monday						
Tuesday						
Wednesday						
Thursday						
Friday						
Saturday						
Sunday						

DATE						
DAY	Breakfast	Lunch	Dinner	Snack	Bedtime	Other
Monday						
Tuesday						
Wednesday						
Thursday						
Friday						
Saturday						
Sunday						

SUGAR MONITOR

DATE						
DAY	Breakfast	Lunch	Dinner	Snack	Bedtime	Other
Monday						
Tuesday						
Wednesday						
Thursday						
Friday						
Saturday						
Sunday						

DATE						
DAY	Breakfast	Lunch	Dinner	Snack	Bedtime	Other
Monday						
Tuesday						
Wednesday						
Thursday						
Friday						
Saturday						
Sunday						

SUGAR MONITOR

DATE						
DAY	Breakfast	Lunch	Dinner	Snack	Bedtime	Other
Monday						
Tuesday						
Wednesday						
Thursday						
Friday						
Saturday						
Sunday						

DATE						
DAY	Breakfast	Lunch	Dinner	Snack	Bedtime	Other
Monday						
Tuesday						
Wednesday						
Thursday						
Friday						
Saturday						
Sunday						

SUGAR MONITOR

DATE						
DAY	Breakfast	Lunch	Dinner	Snack	Bedtime	Other
Monday						
Tuesday						
Wednesday						
Thursday						
Friday						
Saturday						
Sunday						

DATE						
DAY	Breakfast	Lunch	Dinner	Snack	Bedtime	Other
Monday						
Tuesday						
Wednesday						
Thursday						
Friday						
Saturday						
Sunday						

SUGAR MONITOR

DATE						
DAY	Breakfast	Lunch	Dinner	Snack	Bedtime	Other
Monday						
Tuesday						
Wednesday						
Thursday						
Friday						
Saturday						
Sunday						

DATE						
DAY	Breakfast	Lunch	Dinner	Snack	Bedtime	Other
Monday						
Tuesday						
Wednesday						
Thursday						
Friday						
Saturday						
Sunday						

SUGAR MONITOR

DATE						
DAY	Breakfast	Lunch	Dinner	Snack	Bedtime	Other
Monday						
Tuesday						
Wednesday						
Thursday						
Friday						
Saturday						
Sunday						

DATE						
DAY	Breakfast	Lunch	Dinner	Snack	Bedtime	Other
Monday						
Tuesday						
Wednesday						
Thursday						
Friday						
Saturday						
Sunday						

SUGAR MONITOR

DATE						
DAY	Breakfast	Lunch	Dinner	Snack	Bedtime	Other
Monday						
Tuesday						
Wednesday						
Thursday						
Friday						
Saturday						
Sunday						

DATE						
DAY	Breakfast	Lunch	Dinner	Snack	Bedtime	Other
Monday						
Tuesday						
Wednesday						
Thursday						
Friday						
Saturday						
Sunday						

SUGAR MONITOR

DATE						
DAY	Breakfast	Lunch	Dinner	Snack	Bedtime	Other
Monday						
Tuesday						
Wednesday						
Thursday						
Friday						
Saturday						
Sunday						

DATE						
DAY	Breakfast	Lunch	Dinner	Snack	Bedtime	Other
Monday						
Tuesday						
Wednesday						
Thursday						
Friday						
Saturday						
Sunday						

SUGAR MONITOR

DATE						
DAY	Breakfast	Lunch	Dinner	Snack	Bedtime	Other
Monday						
Tuesday						
Wednesday						
Thursday						
Friday						
Saturday						
Sunday						

DATE						
DAY	Breakfast	Lunch	Dinner	Snack	Bedtime	Other
Monday						
Tuesday						
Wednesday						
Thursday						
Friday						
Saturday						
Sunday						

SUGAR MONITOR

DATE						
DAY	Breakfast	Lunch	Dinner	Snack	Bedtime	Other
Monday						
Tuesday						
Wednesday						
Thursday						
Friday						
Saturday						
Sunday						

DATE						
DAY	Breakfast	Lunch	Dinner	Snack	Bedtime	Other
Monday						
Tuesday						
Wednesday						
Thursday						
Friday						
Saturday						
Sunday						

SUGAR MONITOR

DATE						
DAY	Breakfast	Lunch	Dinner	Snack	Bedtime	Other
Monday						
Tuesday						
Wednesday						
Thursday						
Friday						
Saturday						
Sunday						

DATE						
DAY	Breakfast	Lunch	Dinner	Snack	Bedtime	Other
Monday						
Tuesday						
Wednesday						
Thursday						
Friday						
Saturday						
Sunday						

SUGAR MONITOR

DATE						
DAY	Breakfast	Lunch	Dinner	Snack	Bedtime	Other
Monday						
Tuesday						
Wednesday						
Thursday						
Friday						
Saturday						
Sunday						

DATE						
DAY	Breakfast	Lunch	Dinner	Snack	Bedtime	Other
Monday						
Tuesday						
Wednesday						
Thursday						
Friday						
Saturday						
Sunday						

SUGAR MONITOR

DATE						
DAY	Breakfast	Lunch	Dinner	Snack	Bedtime	Other
Monday						
Tuesday						
Wednesday						
Thursday						
Friday						
Saturday						
Sunday						

DATE						
DAY	Breakfast	Lunch	Dinner	Snack	Bedtime	Other
Monday						
Tuesday						
Wednesday						
Thursday						
Friday						
Saturday						
Sunday						

SUGAR MONITOR

DATE						
DAY	Breakfast	Lunch	Dinner	Snack	Bedtime	Other
Monday						
Tuesday						
Wednesday						
Thursday						
Friday						
Saturday						
Sunday						

DATE						
DAY	Breakfast	Lunch	Dinner	Snack	Bedtime	Other
Monday						
Tuesday						
Wednesday						
Thursday						
Friday						
Saturday						
Sunday						

SUGAR MONITOR

DATE						
DAY	Breakfast	Lunch	Dinner	Snack	Bedtime	Other
Monday						
Tuesday						
Wednesday						
Thursday						
Friday						
Saturday						
Sunday						

DATE						
DAY	Breakfast	Lunch	Dinner	Snack	Bedtime	Other
Monday						
Tuesday						
Wednesday						
Thursday						
Friday						
Saturday						
Sunday						

SUGAR MONITOR

DATE						
DAY	Breakfast	Lunch	Dinner	Snack	Bedtime	Other
Monday						
Tuesday						
Wednesday						
Thursday						
Friday						
Saturday						
Sunday						

DATE						
DAY	Breakfast	Lunch	Dinner	Snack	Bedtime	Other
Monday						
Tuesday						
Wednesday						
Thursday						
Friday						
Saturday						
Sunday						

SUGAR MONITOR

DATE						
DAY	Breakfast	Lunch	Dinner	Snack	Bedtime	Other
Monday						
Tuesday						
Wednesday						
Thursday						
Friday						
Saturday						
Sunday						

DATE						
DAY	Breakfast	Lunch	Dinner	Snack	Bedtime	Other
Monday						
Tuesday						
Wednesday						
Thursday						
Friday						
Saturday						
Sunday						

SUGAR MONITOR

DATE						
DAY	Breakfast	Lunch	Dinner	Snack	Bedtime	Other
Monday						
Tuesday						
Wednesday						
Thursday						
Friday						
Saturday						
Sunday						

DATE						
DAY	Breakfast	Lunch	Dinner	Snack	Bedtime	Other
Monday						
Tuesday						
Wednesday						
Thursday						
Friday						
Saturday						
Sunday						

SUGAR MONITOR

DATE						
DAY	Breakfast	Lunch	Dinner	Snack	Bedtime	Other
Monday						
Tuesday						
Wednesday						
Thursday						
Friday						
Saturday						
Sunday						

DATE						
DAY	Breakfast	Lunch	Dinner	Snack	Bedtime	Other
Monday						
Tuesday						
Wednesday						
Thursday						
Friday						
Saturday						
Sunday						

SUGAR MONITOR

DATE						
DAY	Breakfast	Lunch	Dinner	Snack	Bedtime	Other
Monday						
Tuesday						
Wednesday						
Thursday						
Friday						
Saturday						
Sunday						

DATE						
DAY	Breakfast	Lunch	Dinner	Snack	Bedtime	Other
Monday						
Tuesday						
Wednesday						
Thursday						
Friday						
Saturday						
Sunday						

SUGAR MONITOR

DATE						
DAY	Breakfast	Lunch	Dinner	Snack	Bedtime	Other
Monday						
Tuesday						
Wednesday						
Thursday						
Friday						
Saturday						
Sunday						

DATE						
DAY	Breakfast	Lunch	Dinner	Snack	Bedtime	Other
Monday						
Tuesday						
Wednesday						
Thursday						
Friday						
Saturday						
Sunday						

SUGAR MONITOR

DATE						
DAY	Breakfast	Lunch	Dinner	Snack	Bedtime	Other
Monday						
Tuesday						
Wednesday						
Thursday						
Friday						
Saturday						
Sunday						

DATE						
DAY	Breakfast	Lunch	Dinner	Snack	Bedtime	Other
Monday						
Tuesday						
Wednesday						
Thursday						
Friday						
Saturday						
Sunday						

SUGAR MONITOR

DATE						
DAY	Breakfast	Lunch	Dinner	Snack	Bedtime	Other
Monday						
Tuesday						
Wednesday						
Thursday						
Friday						
Saturday						
Sunday						

DATE						
DAY	Breakfast	Lunch	Dinner	Snack	Bedtime	Other
Monday						
Tuesday						
Wednesday						
Thursday						
Friday						
Saturday						
Sunday						

SUGAR MONITOR

DATE						
DAY	Breakfast	Lunch	Dinner	Snack	Bedtime	Other
Monday						
Tuesday						
Wednesday						
Thursday						
Friday						
Saturday						
Sunday						

DATE						
DAY	Breakfast	Lunch	Dinner	Snack	Bedtime	Other
Monday						
Tuesday						
Wednesday						
Thursday						
Friday						
Saturday						
Sunday						

SUGAR MONITOR

DATE						
DAY	Breakfast	Lunch	Dinner	Snack	Bedtime	Other
Monday						
Tuesday						
Wednesday						
Thursday						
Friday						
Saturday						
Sunday						

DATE						
DAY	Breakfast	Lunch	Dinner	Snack	Bedtime	Other
Monday						
Tuesday						
Wednesday						
Thursday						
Friday						
Saturday						
Sunday						

SUGAR MONITOR

DATE						
DAY	Breakfast	Lunch	Dinner	Snack	Bedtime	Other
Monday						
Tuesday						
Wednesday						
Thursday						
Friday						
Saturday						
Sunday						

DATE						
DAY	Breakfast	Lunch	Dinner	Snack	Bedtime	Other
Monday						
Tuesday						
Wednesday						
Thursday						
Friday						
Saturday						
Sunday						

SUGAR MONITOR

DATE						
DAY	Breakfast	Lunch	Dinner	Snack	Bedtime	Other
Monday						
Tuesday						
Wednesday						
Thursday						
Friday						
Saturday						
Sunday						

DATE						
DAY	Breakfast	Lunch	Dinner	Snack	Bedtime	Other
Monday						
Tuesday						
Wednesday						
Thursday						
Friday						
Saturday						
Sunday						

NOTE

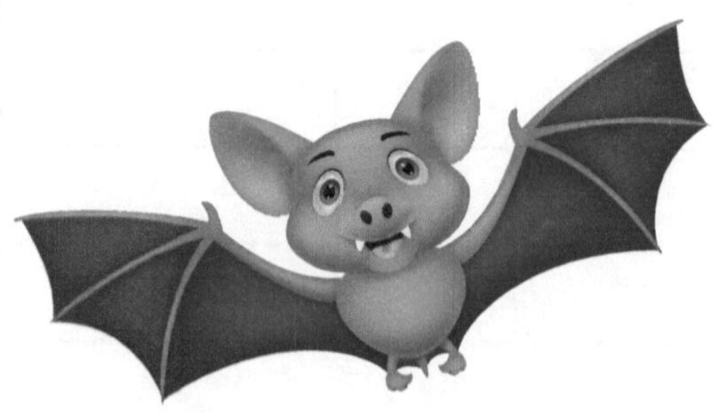

NOTE

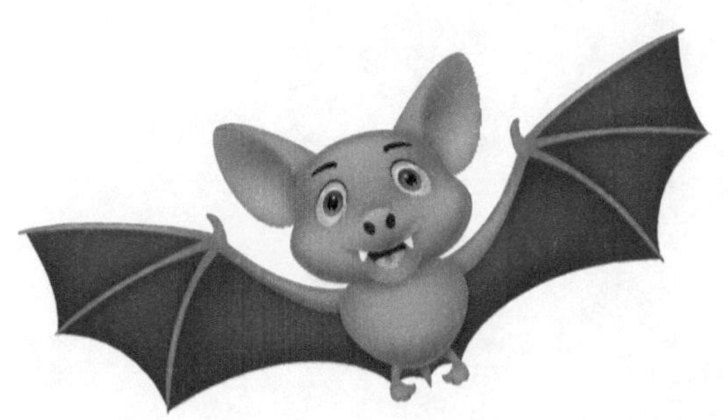

www.ingramcontent.com/pod-product-compliance
Lightning Source LLC
Chambersburg PA
CBHW031300250726
48655CB00005B/2286